7 Day Green Juice Detox

Natalia Krasnyanskaya
and the editors of top.me

ISBN: 1503098036
ISBN-13: 978-1503098039

MEDICAL ADVICE DISCLAIMER

CONTENTS

FURTHER READING

Please follow us for daily health and fitness advice, tips and tricks, tasty recipes and more on:
www.top.me

INTRODUCTION

Congratulations on taking the first steps to get to a healthier lifestyle. Green juices are a great source of vitamins, nutrition and craving cutting goodness! Once you start doing the method outlined inside this book you will find yourself with more energy, healthier skin, a large amount of confidence and the need to snack nearly removed from your lifestyle completely.

That is just what drinking green juices is all about! Honestly, so few people understand the true power of greens and many people dislike drinking them because of their odd look. While they may look odd being juiced the flavor and benefits are much better than anyone can image.

Instead of having to take that huge multivitamin each and every day, you can complete the 7 day detox method outlined in this book and get those same benefits. Greens juices provide you with a way to get all the needed vitamins you should be eating daily. Green vegetables contain calcium, iron, magnesium, vitamins A, C, K and a ton of B vitamins as well. You can get a lot more energy from a 6 oz glass of green juice then you can from a 16 oz mug of coffee. The best part is that green juices cut craving and give you a full feeling faster and longer than any other item.

To your health!
Natalia Krasnyanskaya
Editor in Chief, Top.me

☐

THE MANY BENEFITS OF GREEN JUICE DETOXING

Tastes Great

Once you start drinking green juices offer you will learn that you don't really taste the greens in the juice when they are combined with a nice amount of sweet and healthy fruits. This is because most greens are tasteless. Spinach for example may have a strong taste when cooked but when it's added to fruits like oranges, peaches and even apples you won't even taste the spinach.

Gives Energy

Once you start drinking green juices you will feel an amount of energy that will last all day long. This is because of the B vitamins within the greens. Many times people drink coffee or energy drinks to wake them up. The truth is that a surge from coffee or energy drink is very short lived.

Boost Metabolism

Once you start drinking green juices you will learn a unique way to manage your health, start a diet and completely clean your body of gross toxins. This detoxing method can be used to start a diet because it remove the toxins that might be living in your body currently. You will notice you are no longer constipated and have no problem going to the bathroom each and every night during the time you are doing the seven day green juice diet.

The Importance of Phytonutrients

Now you know of all benefits of juicing. But what is so vital in fruits and vegetables that helps us to stay healthy? The answer is phytonutrients or phytochemicals. These are chemical compounds that occur naturally in plants (phyto means "plant" in Greek). There are over 10,000 known phytonutrients, and the best part about it is scientists are discovering more and more all the time. These nutrients are what give fruit and vegetables their intense color and phenomenal nutrition.

Fruits and vegetables consist of hundreds of different phytonutrients that protect the body from disease. No single fruit or vegetable can provide every beneficial chemical, so eating or drinking juice from a variety of colourful foods is key.

- Phytonutrients may:
- serve as antioxidants
- enhance immune response
- enhance cell-to-cell communication
- alter estrogen metabolism

- convert to vitamin A (beta-carotene is metabolized to vitamin A)
- cause cancer cells to die (apoptosis)
- repair DNA damage caused by smoking and other toxic exposures
- detoxify carcinogens

Phytonutrients are usually most beneficial when consumed in raw foods as when you cook veggies or process the natural state of the plant, you kill most of the phytonutrients.

This is why juicing is such a good way to consume your fruits and veggies. You keep them in a raw state, but just turn them from solids to liquids.

There are over 10,000 known phytonutrients, and the best part about it is scientists are discovering more and more all the time. These nutrients are what give fruit and vegetables their intense color and phenomenal nutrition.

The major classes of phytonutrients include:

- Organo-sulfurs: the glucobrassins found in crucifers and the allyl sulfur compounds in garlic.
- Terpenoids: include the basic terpenoids like limonene found in citrus foods and menthol, as well as the carotenoids (vitamin A), coenzyme Q10, the phytosterols, and the tocopherols and tocotrienols.
- Flavonoids: the plant pigments that give plants their colors, like the deep blue of blueberries, the purple of grapes, the orange of pumpkins, or the red of tomatoes. Flavonoids include the anthocyanidins in blueberries and quercetin found in onions.
- Isoflavonoids and lignans: For example, genistein and diadzein found in soy foods, and the lignans in flaxseed and rye.
- Organic acids: ferulic acid, which is found in whole grains, and the coumarins, which are found in parsely, licorice and citrus fruits.

Phytonutrients in Fruits

Anthocyanidins are the purple-blue pigments that give fruits such as blueberries, blackberries, raspberries, black currants, and red and purple grapes their unique coloration, and which protect them from the damaging effects of oxidation. These phytonutrients not only support the health of plants, but can support the health of humans as well.

Among the antioxidants, anthocyanidins have been found to have some unique features. They are able to protect cells and tissues from free radical damage in both water-soluble and fat-soluble environments.

Phytochemicals in Vegetables

The foods we loved to hate as kids have turned out to be especially healthy for us. Members of the brassica family of vegetables, including broccoli, Brussels sprouts, cabbage, kale and bok choy appear to have significant cancer-preventive properties.

In plants, glucosinolates react with an enzyme called myrosinase that converts them into related compounds known as indoles and isothiocyanates. These phytochemicals seem to reduce the potential of carcinogens through their ability to beneficially modulate liver detoxification enzymes — they inhibit certain enzymes that normally activate carcinogens while also inducing other enzymes that help to dismantle active carcinogens.

About 10% of the population consumes less than one serving of vegetable per day and about 48% consume less than one serving of fruit a day.

Juicing is a great way to mix different fruits and vegetables as daily you have to consume at least five servings of high quality fruits and vegetables. Juicing make it much easier as you have many different phytochemicals in one glass.

PREPARING FOR JUICING

Of course with everything good there are always some bad things that come with them. While green juices provide more positive things than negative ones it's important for you to know right away what the negatives might be and how to cope with them.

The first problem is that it does cost to do a detox. You must be willing to buy the ingredients in order to even begin. You also need to be able to buy a juicer that is long lasting and can provide you with the features you need

Of course the cost of ingredients depends on you and how you shop - but it can get expensive. You should budget for an extra $20 to $45 for your seven day detox because of the things you will need.

Normally you can spend anywhere from $20 to $200 on a juicer. The investment is worth it because more expensive juicers last for years while cheaper ones might need to be replaced after a few months of steady juicing. It's not recommended to use a blender when it comes to this detox method. You want to juice the ingredients to get the most nutrients out of them instead of just blending them into mush.

The second problem is that dieting of any kind is hard and so is detoxing. It takes times and patience to get started and to last for the whole seven days.

The good news is that this detox lasts only for 7 days! Of course, you can repeat it as often as you like, for example monthly, but a 7 day spread is much easier to do than a longer diet.

☐

HOW TO CHOOSE A JUICER

Are you ready for your green juice detox? Finally! But of course buying a home juicer isn't as easy as it may sound at first. There are so many juicers to choose from and once you see a few of them they all start to look the same.

Masticating Juicer vs Centrifugal Juicers

There are two different types of juicers. One is called Masticating and the other is called Centrifugal.

There are also juicers that have do a mixture of both. Both centrifugal and masticating have their own unique pros and cons but generally masticating juicers tend to be quieter than centrifugal juicers, while centrifugal normally work a lot faster.

It's important to consider what kind of vegetables and fruits you will be juicing. This is because some fruits and vegetables won't produce enough juice when compared to others. If you are planning on doing a lot of leafy vegetables such as spinach, kale or wheat grass, a masticating juicer normally will produce a lot more juice without having to use a lot of the vegetable. However, if you are planning to add a lot of different varieties of fruits and vegetables, a centrifugal juicer will produce for a more evenly blend.

Another important thing to consider is clean up. Juicers require cleaning just like any other kitchen appliance. However, some juicers are much harder to clean than others. Centrifugal juicers normally require more thorough cleaning when compared to masticating juicers. Masticating juicers normally just require removal of the veggies' remnants and good rinse.

Lastly, consider your price point. Just because a juicer cost a lot of money doesn't mean it's going to fit all your requirements. Consider what you are hoping to make and how often you are really planning on using it.

Masticating Juicer Pros and Cons

Pros
- Better at extracting juice than centrifugal juicers. Higher juice yield.
- Very good at juicing leafy green vegetables.
- Higher nutritional value due to slow speed mastication.
- Can be used for other tasks (coffee grinding, herb mincing, baby food preparation, etc).
- Juice has less foam.
- Less noisy. Due to the slow grinding motors, the noise level is very low.
- Longer shelf life. Because there is no oxidation, juice can be kept for more than 72 hours.

Cons
- Slow. Takes longer to juice than centrifugal juicers.
- More expensive. Prices can be much higher than centrifugal juicers.
- Needs more effort. Fruit and vegetables must be chopped into smaller manageable chunks before juicing.
- More bulky. Their larger lie flat design occupies more counter space.

Centrifugal Juicers – Pros and Cons

Pros
- Fast juicing.
- Easy to clean. Dishwasher safe.
- Handles large fruit chunks easily.
- Compact vertical design takes less counter space.
- Cheaper than masticating juicers.
- Excellent for busy, large families, or even events or parties.

Cons
- Bad with leafy greens and wheat grass.
- Extracts less juice than masticating juicers.
- Less nutritional value. High speed and speed affects the quality of the juice.
- Produce more foam.
- Higher noise level. The high speed motor results in more noise.
- Shorter juice lifespan. Juice from centrifugal machines cannot be kept for long. Needs to be consumed immediately.□

11 WAYS TO INCLUDE JUICING IN YOUR DIET

If you're going to start a juicing diet, it may be helpful to start with a few days of eating primarily fruits and vegetables before going over to all-juice. This helps reduce dependence on sugar, flour, and other common diet staples that can make a juice diet difficult to swallow.

For those who are ready to start your juicing, here are some useful tips of how to do it easily:

The Freshest, the Best

When making the juice, make absolutely sure to get fresh, healthy fruits. Look for produce that have a full color, are firm to the touch, and have green, leafy tops. Avoid fruits with the following signs:
- rubberiness
- limpness
- wilted tops
- excessive cracking

Mix in Vegetables

Try vegetables mixed with your favorite fruits in your juicer. Many vegetables are easy to juice. They can add important vitamins and minerals to your juice as well. In addition, using vegetables can cut down on the calorie count of your juice, which in turn, makes it a better diet option.

Vegetables that you do not like alone might end up tasting great to you when mixed in a juice with other flavors. This is a great way to get nutrients you otherwise wouldn't.

Never add more than one new vegetable to your juice mix at a time. If you do not like the taste of the juice, or your digestive system does not react well to your new juice blend, you will not know what vegetable to reduce or avoid if you add a bunch of new veggies in the same batch.

Juicing vegetables allows you to quickly and easily get the most nutrients out of them that you possibly can without spending a ton of time on them.

Making healthy juice from vegetables is wonderful, however, do not go overboard with variety. Stick to using 2-3 vegetables in your juice blends and incorporate apple into the mix. You will minimize the amount of flavors you are trying to combine and the apple will add the right amount of sweet to the mix for extra enjoyment.

Freeze Some For "Rainy Days"

Juicing is a lifestyle you dedicate yourself to, and you will notice if you miss a day. So if you're not able to buy some fresh fruits for your juice, keep some in the freezer or even freeze some juice to tide you over.

Store the Juice Right

If you must store your juice in the fridge, add a tablespoon of lemon juice. It shouldn't have a major effect on the flavor, but it will keep the juice from becoming discolored as it sits, creating a more appetizing effect. Always try to make your juice just before you drink it, for maximum health benefits.

Choose a container that is airtight. Label your juice so that you remember what you are drinking, and enjoy!

Remember:

Healthy juice is best at room temperature, so make sure to take the produce out of the fridge for a little while before you make the juice. Drinking cold juice can shut slow down the digestive system.

Buy Fruits in Bulk

Go to local farms with your friends or family and purchase in bulk to get larger discounts. Many items can be kept in a cool, dark place for longer periods of time. Apple farms, for example, will sell you bushel after bushel for decreasing costs per pound. So, load the back with apples, and share with everyone! They don't have to be juicers to enjoy fresh produce.

Though, don't buy too many fruits and vegetables at a time that spoil quickly. You might end up buying much more than you will use, and the extra food will decay and go to waste. Experiment with different amounts to see how much juice you drink a day, so you know how much produce you have to buy in advance.

Safe For Diabetic

Are you diabetic? Juicing can still be for you! You can juice so many different items that you'll always be able to have a selection that does not contain too many carbohydrates or a large dose of sugar. You can also include milk or yogurt in your drink to up your dairy intake.

Chill Out

What a tasty and quick way to chill out trying adding chopped ice to your juice to make it a cool treat in the summer! It's like drinking a smoothie.

Bananas and papayas do not seem to do well in a juicer. You can still use them with juice, but it is best to stick them in a blender. They are very thick, and tend to work better when making fruit smoothies or any type of frozen dessert that you make.

Make It Smooth

If you want your juice to be very smooth and free of pulp, try using a coffee filter or cheese cloth to strain it after it comes out of the juicer. Also keep in mind that the softer the produce used, the thicker the juice tends to be for example, tomato juice.

Make It a Habit

If you are trying to make sure you stick with your healthy new juicing habit, make sure that the juice machine stays on your kitchen counter at all times. Out of sight, out of mind is especially true when it comes to trying to form new habits. By making sure your juicer is always in plain sight, you will be more likely to remember to use it every day.

Add New Flavors

Wheat-grass has many health benefits such as cleansing the lymph system, and removing toxic metals from your cells. You can only ingest wheat-grass through juice, so juicing can be extremely beneficial. Be careful because wheat-grass does have a very strong taste. It is best to start out a little at a time. Each time you juice, just gradually add a little more.

Try wheatgrass with apple/ginger/orange juice, but you can come up with a hundred more recipes. Give it a try.

Get adventurous with your juicing ingredients! Why not try grapefruit or add in a little ginger for some zip! Other items to try are celery, parsley, beets, bell peppers, and leafy greens! You never know what you might end up liking.

Try spices like cayenne or cinnamon, or nutrition-packed additions like spirulina. You can even put a little honey and yogurt in once in a while for a sweet, smooth treat. Make sure to use only non-fat, unsweetened dairy to keep the resulting produce healthy.

There are a million-and-one recipes of items to include in your juicer. How about a combination like apple with carrot and ginger, or celery and pear. My favorites are apple with lemon and pear, apple with cinnamon and honey, and banana with mango and orange. Try new ideas to find your own favorites!

If you're making carrot juice, here's a little tip to give it a better, more interesting flavor. Try adding cilantro! It has a nice, refreshing, satisfying aspect that compliments the sweetness of carrot juice.

Buy Local

Try to use locally-grown fruits and vegetables in your juicing. The best option is to use produce that you've grown yourself. Every mile that a piece of fruit needs to be transported to get to you increases the carbon footprint of your glass of juice. It also increases the chance of your produce becoming contaminated with bacteria or chemicals.

Buying fruit and vegetables for your juicing can be easy by using all five senses to find the freshest produce to bring home. Sniff the item and make sure it smells good, like you would want to eat it. Squeeze it and feel if it's too hard or too soft. Look it over for imperfections, and then take it home and taste a bit.

Save Your Money

You don't have to spend a fortune on fresh juicing produce as long as you shop in season. Berries are great in the summer, but will cost you an arm and a leg to buy in the winter, so skip them until the prices drop again. Apples last all winter, so feel free to buy a few bushels and keep them in the garage.

Add Fats

Fats are still important while juicing. Nuts and seeds contain not only necessary fats but proteins as well. Blending nuts and seeds with your juices will give the juice extra protein, necessary amino acids which help the immune system and the brain and the good types of fat your body needs.

Research Before Juicing

Before you get started juicing, do a little bit of research on the different varieties of fruits and veggies available. There are a lot of variances in the nutrients that are found in each of the fruits and veggies. Your best option is to mix items that will provide you with a variety of vitamins and minerals, ones that will meet your daily requirements. You will not just be supplying your body with proper nutrients, but you are going to find some very interesting blends.

Get Rid of All Harmful

Remove pits and seeds from your fruits before juicing them. Hard pits, like those found in peaches, will leave unpleasant chunks in your juice and can damage the blades of your juicer. Other seeds, such as apple seeds, may actually contain chemicals that are harmful. It's best to remove them beforehand.

Health Benefits by Juice Mix

Health Benefits	Fruit and Vegetable Mixes
Boost and cleanse our system	Carrot-Ginger-Apple
Prevent cancer, reduce cholesterol, and improve stomach upset and headache	Apple-Cucumber-Celery
Improve skin complexion and stops bad breath	Tomato-Carrot-Apple
Avoid bad breath and reduce internal body heat	Bitter Gourd-Apple-Milk
Improve Skin texture and moisture and reduce body heat	Orange-Ginger-Cucumber
To dispel excess salts, nourish the bladder and kidney	Pineapple-Apple-Watermelon
To improve skin complexion	Apple-Cucumber-Kiwi
To regulate sugar content	Pear-Banana
Clear body heat, counteract toxicity, decrease blood pressure and fight oxidization	Carrot-Apple-Pear-Mango
Rich in Vitamin C & Vitamin B2 that increase cell activity and strengthen body immunity	Honeydew-Grape-Watermelon-Milk
Rich in Vitamin C, E, and Iron. Improve skin complexion and metabolism	Papaya-Pineapple-Milk
Rich in vitamin, it prevents constipation	Banana-Pineapple-Milk

GETTING STARTED WITH THE DETOX

Before we get to the step by step method, here are some tips that can help you get the most out of this detox method.

• Tip 1 – Keep a positive mind set every time you make and drink your juice. It's very important to think of the end result while in the process of the method.

• Tip 2 – Lower the amount of carbs you eat. Some detoxing diets advise you to remove carbs from your diet completely but you don't have to with this detox diet. Instead cut your carbs in half and eat everything like normally.

• Tip 3 – Don't eat sweets or salty items. This can ruin this detoxing completely. Instead of eating a piece of cake from the office party, eat some yogurt instead. This will give you a sweet flavor without the high amount of sugar. The same goes for chips and other salty things.

• Tip 4 – Drink lots of water and cut out the soda. Even diet sodas are not good during this detox.

• Tip 5 – Get active. You don't have to change your whole life in order to get active while detoxing your body. Take the stairs to work instead of the elevator. Go for a walk in the park. The detox gives you the energy to do it.

• Tip 6 – Plan a way to celebrate after you've completed the detoxing diet. This reward should not be food, it should be something fun and something that you are looking forward to.

POSSIBLE SIDE EFFECTS OF JUICING

Juicing is a great way to clean your body, fight disease and stay healthy. Though, beyond all the benefits that juicing provides, there are some potential serious side effects. Most of them are temporary. If any other symptoms occur, consult your doctor.

Possible side effects:

- Fluctuation of energy levels
- Dizziness
- Headache
- Drop in muscle mass, which leads to physical weakness and fatigue.
- Diarrhea or constipation
- Increased body oder or bad breath
- Carotenemia, a condition that causes discoloration of the skin when too many orange vegetables are consumed
- Dehydration and paleness

If you experience fainting, extreme dizziness, low blood pressure, vomiting, severe diarrhea, stop your juicing and contact your physician. With some adjustments to your detox plan most side effects can often be resolved.

DETOX STEP BY STEP
1 – Pick Your Recipes

Start with 2 to 3 for the first 7 days. The great thing about green juicing is that it's easy to blend the flavors with greens without even noticing them. Your body will notice but your taste buds will just taste the main things.

2 – Get a Juicer

Buy a great juicer if you don't have one and buy your ingredients.

3 – Plan Ahead

Plan your juice drinking times for breakfast or lunch, not dinner.

4 – Prepare Your Ingredients

Prep your ingredients by chopping and placing them into serving sized bags the day before juicing. This will save you time. Freeze the goodies in an air tight bag and take them out 2 to 3 hours before juicing them.

5 – Drink It!

Drink your juice 30 minutes before eating a meal- This will provide you with a nice filling feeling and help to reduce serving sizes.

6 – Cut The Eating

Cut your meal in half and eat little to no carbs within each meal. Avoid sweets and also coffee while you are on this detox.

7 – Be Active

Get fit and stay active. Normally after drinking your juice and eating a meal you will notice a burst of energy. Take advantage of this and get active.

8 – Just 7 Days

Do this for seven days. Normally after two days it becomes a normal thing and doesn't seem difficult any longer.

9 – Ease Out

After seven days, go back to eating normally but still cut back on your carbs for two more days and continue exercising. Don't be surprised if you notice your energy lower once you stop drinking green juices. This is a normal thing and normally goes away after you go back to your normal routine. Keep away from coffee for 2 days after the seven days. Many times coffee can reverse the detoxing so take a coffee break and drink tea instead.

HOW TO EAT AFTER THE DETOX

Don't just slip back to your old eating habits! Now is the time to re-evaluate and reset your diet.

There are two good options how to eat after a fast. The first one is to slowly incorporate solid food back into your everyday eating. It's easy to start with one meal a day for the first three days and then work your way up to 2-3 meals over the course of a week. I would suggest eating fresh fruits and veggies for the first three days. You basically want to eat the same stuff you have been juicing. After three days you should be safe to add a protein, such as a chicken breast, steak, pork chop, tuna, etc. This will slowly introduce solids back into your system and ensure you don't fall back on to bad habits.

The second option is to eat only fresh fruits and vegetables for a complete week after your detox. This gives your body time to adjust to solids over liquid, and since you are eating the same thing you are juicing, your body will adjust pretty faster.

Do's and Don'ts

Once you decide how to eat after your detox, there are a few do's and don'ts that you should keep in mind.

Here are a few things to avoid in the first week after the detox: soda, alcohol, candy or sweets, dairy, and breads. In choosing not to eat or drink anything on that list for the first week off my fast, you are setting the pace for the new habits you will develop in your diet.

After you come off your detox and start eating solids, make a conscious decision to avoid snacking. Eating different snacks between main meals can cause you to drift right back into other bad habits, and we don't want that to happen.

The second you should do is to come up with a meal plan. This is a great time for a critical look at your diet.

Make sure you are limiting yourself to 4 to 6 meals per day. Meal sizes should be about the size of one and a half of your fists. You can have juices while you are incorporating solids back into your diet. You will be surprised at how you will start to crave your juices more after you go back to solids.

29 TASTY JUICE RECIPES

Tropical Veggie

1 cucumber peeled
1 cup pineapple peeled

Greens with Carrots

6 carrots
1 inch of fresh ginger
1handful fresh greens

Pine -Berries

10 ripe strawberries
1 cup pineapple peals.

Just Veggies

2 beet greens
4 broccoli spears
1 cup cauliflower
1 handful fresh greens
1 piece of ginger

Apple-Papaya

1 red apple cored
1 small papaya seeds included
1 medium orange peeled

Sweet Greens

2 yellow apples cored
1 stalk of celery
1 handful parsley
2 handfuls of spinach
5 leaves of iceberg lettuce

Lemony- Apple

2 green apple cored
1 lemon peeled
1 orange peels

Vitamin Orange

4 oranges peeled
2 cups of pineapple peeled
1 small sweet potato

Quick Tropical

2 apples cored

3 kiwis not peeled
4 ripe pears cored

Orange Spring Time

1 apple peeled and cored
2 ripe pears cored
2 oranges peeled

Tangy Apple

5 apples cored
1 lemon peeled

Green Country

5 roman tomatoes
handful of spinach

Tangy Carrot Juice

5 carrots
1 apple
½ peeled cucumber
1 beet
1 stalk celery
2 pieces of fresh ginger

Easy Three

1 medium cucumber with skin
1 carrot
½ red apple

Just The Green

2 stalks of celery
4 stalks of bok choy
2 handfuls of spinach
½ bunch of parsley

Apple Pie Juice

3 granny smith apples cored
1 lemon peeled
1 tsp cinnamon
1 inch piece of ginger

Sparkling Citrus Apple

1 lime
1 lemon
1 apple cored
1 cup sparkling water added after others are juiced.

Sweeter Yams

1 small peeled yam
2 green apples
5 baby carrots

Red and Orange

1 large red apple
5 fresh strawberries
1 orange peeled

Sweet Greens

1 large apple
1 large peach
2 handful of greens

Red Tropical

1 large peach
5 fresh strawberries
1 nectarine pitted
1 mango pitted and skin removed
1 pear

Summer Yummy

2 peaches with seeds removed
1 nectarine pitted
1 lemon peeled

Long and Tasty

1 kiwi
1 mango pitted and skin removed
1 radish
1 pear
1 radish
1 handful of greens
1 handful of spinach
1 bell pepper
1 lemon peeled
1 green apple

Kickin' Sweetness

1 container of blackberries
1 lemon peeled
1 container of raspberries
2 pieces of ginger
1 teaspoon of hot sauce

Asian Pleasure

2 asian pears
1 handful of parsley
1 lemon peeled
¼ cup wheat grass

Spring Yummy

1 carrot peeled
1 handful of spinach
1 asian pear
 cup watermelon cups

Pink Ice

1 banana
5 strawberries
1/2 grapefruit
1/2 orange

Mixed Fruit Explosion

1 banana
1 kiwi
1/2 mango
1/2 papaya
1/2 orange

Happy Drink

1 banana
1 kiwi
1 orange

SIX MAGICAL SEEDS THAT WILL BOOST YOUR HEALTH

Juicing helps to boost your metabolism. After your detox, add some of these magic seeds to your diet. They contain valuable micronutrients like folic acid and iron and are a great source of dietary fiber.

Chia Seeds

These poppy-like seeds is favorite among many people not only because of the variety of micronutrients it holds, but also because of its property of absorbing the liquid you place it in. It forms a gel around each seed, giving it a pomegranate-like texture. Research shows that it is chock full of lipid antioxidants, which can help prevent cancer, proteins, poly-unsaturated fatty acids (PUFAs), and dietary fiber.

Chia seeds can be mixed with cereal, or you can just let them soak with almond milk for about 15 minutes and then add a little honey or sugar. Because they are so small, you can add them to your salads or any baked recipe you make!

Amaranth Seeds

While they have been classified as "grains" because of their texture after they have been air-puffed, they are technically seeds since they do not come from a cereal plan. These seeds, which are native to the Americas, have a good amount of highly-digestible protein, and linoleic acid which essential for human nutrition. In addition, it is high in iron which will help you prevent having an anemia.

Amaranth tastes and feels almost like tiny pieces of popcorn, and you might enjoy eating it just as is! It is also good on cereal, and terrific in smoothies.

Hemp Seeds

Hemp seeds are full of PUFAs which have been noted to have great anti-inflammatory properties and it's ability to raise metabolic rates. This seed has a special component called Cannabidiol (CBD), which has antimicrobial and anti-convulsive properties, as well as anti-allergenic properties.

The easiest way to take advantage of the nutritional benefits of hemp seeds is by buying hempseed oil. However, the seeds can be found in their full form at health food stores.

Flax Seeds

This tiny seed is thankfully commonly found in 100% multigrain breads and some whole-gran cereals. Each of these tiny seeds have incredibly powerful nutritional properties, ranging from reducing cholesterol levels in the blood, to slowing mammary tumor growth due to it's lignin and oil components.

Because of the press providing a lot of information about this seed, it is now easily found in supermarkets in its powdered form. You may like sprinkling it on salads, putting in sauces and soups, and even in pastries. When you cook for my family, you can slip it in almost every dish and they won't even notice. It is great for adding nutrition to food for picky eaters.

Pumpkin Seeds

If you tend to munch on things subconsciously when your mind is whirring along, this is a great thing to keep in your bag or in your car. They are a good source of B vitamins, zinc and protein (amino acids). Pumpkin seeds have specific form of protein called tryptophan that has even been shown to be effective in treating social anxiety disorders.

Sunflower Seeds

One of the more well-known and cheaper super-seed options is the Sunflower seeds. Their nutritional properties have been taken advantage of by all food industries. It has lots of protein and vitamin B which are beneficial for women of all ages, particularly pregnant women. They are also a good source of vegetable protein and omega-3 fatty acids. Unlike some plant-foods, sunflower seeds don't contain anti-nutritive properties, or toxical compounds, which means your body can fully take advantage of the nutrients found in the seeds.

In each of these little seeds lies powerful nutritional properties we'd be nuts not to take advantage of.

GOJI BERRIES - FRUIT OF IMMORTALITY

Goji berries grow on bushes that are as high as one to three meters as ovoid fleshy berries during the fall season. They are shriveled, red berries closely resembling red raisins; however, their color is a deeper red. They fall in the category of dry fruits and are tiny in size.

- This super fruit is:
- full of anti-oxidants and Vitamin C, therefore helps to boost your immune system,
- loaded with beta-carotene, which helps promote healthy skin,
- improving eyesight, thanks to a compound called zeaxanthin,
- regulating the concentration of cholesterols, leading to better heart health,
- beneficial for treating male infertility,
- able to improve mood, and even to
- protect against age-related diseases such as Alzheimer's.

Forms of Goji Berries

Goji berries come in several forms such as raw, dried and powdered or seeds.

Goji Berries Seeds

The Goji berry seeds vary according to the region of cultivation and their size. Usually, Goji berries consist of 10-60 very tiny yellow seeds that lie compressed with the embryo.

Dried Goji Berries – the Best Nutritional Value

Dried Goji berries, just like any other dried fruit, have higher nutritional value than their regular version. The high content of bioactive ingredients in dried Goji berries enhances their medicinal and dietary qualities. Dried Goji berries are just deprived of moisture and still contain all nutritional content. This makes them high in sugar and calories, which may be harmful if over-eaten.

Fresh Goji Berries – Rich in Vitamin C

Fresh and raw Goji berries are less popular because of their delicate nature. They contain higher content of Vitamin C compared to dried Goji berries.

Powdered Goji Berries – Let You Be Creative

Goji berries powder has become increasingly popular. This is because it can be mixed with water to make Goji juice. The powder is also easier to blend with other fruits to create smoothies or juices.

A couple of teaspoons can also be used with hot beverages such as tea a to give them an antioxidant boost.

Or sprinkle Goji powder onto desserts, Muesli or yoghurts.

Goji Berries Extracts

The increasing popularity of Goji berries has flooded the markets with Goji berries extracts and supplements for daily use.

Goji berries extract supplements are found as regular powder and in capsules.

How to Select the Best Goji Berries

If you are looking for the perfect Goji berries, make sure you know the following important features:

The area where Goji berries are extensively found is known as the Goji belt. In this region, Goji berries are classified in four different grades. According to the descending order of quality they are named as:

- Super
- King
- Special
- Grade A

The most famous and expensive of these grades is "super". As compared to the lowest quality berries; "grade A", Goji berries categorized as "super" are 41% more expensive.

To fall under the "super" category, there have to be about 240 berries per 50 grams whereas there are about 480 berries per 50 grams in the "grade A" category.

The best berries are grown on the longest planted bushes. The older the bushes, the better the quality of Goji berries. This is because longer established bushes also yield larger berries.

The dryness of Goji berries plays an integral part in their quality. The most optimized dryness results in Goji berries with only 10% of moisture content.

Drier Goji berries are better to consume due to the following reasons:

- When soaked in water, they readily plump up.
- Using them with soups and cereals is easier because they soften quickly.
- They can be easily stored.

THREE VEGETARIAN FOODS YOU SHOULD TRY

When you finish your detox, one of the most important things is going back to your normal eating habits. It's the best time to reconsider your old diet. About the healthy ways of how to come back to your normal eating, read in the chapter "How to eat after detox".

In this chapter we have three tasty foods for you that will make your after detox days easier and diverse. Just try them in your new diet.

Quinoa

Quinoa, which is pronounced as KEEN-wah, is like a grain and a seed at the same time and it is known as a pseudocereal. The seeds that grow on the quinoa plant are actually quite high in starch. These seeds need to be highly processed and manipulated to become a grain substitute.

Most whole grains, when unprocessed, are good for some carbohydrates and a smattering of B vitamins. This is not the case with quinoa. The reason why quinoa is considered as a vegetarian food is because it is high in amino acids, particularly lysine. This means that you can get from this food the same stuff you get from steak. What makes it better though, is that it doesn't have the high fat content and it can actually help lower your cholesterol.

Quinoa also tastes great. Tons of quinoa recipes can be found on the internet, and you can even get it in flour form. You can bake your own quinoa concoctions and reap the benefits of the amino acids without the fat. Even if you don't keep to a strict vegetarian diet you should think about incorporating quinoa in your diet to improve your health.

Seaweed

Seaweed is actually considered quite a delicacy in regions where it is difficult to grow vegetables. For instance, Japan is big into seaweed because they don't have much arable land, and they are surrounded by the ocean where seaweed is abundant.

Soups, salads, and mixed greens are all great places to add seaweed into your diet. Yes, you do need to eat your vegetables – but mix in seaweed to get some different nutrients and break the cycle of broccoli and string beans.

Seaweed has a great number of advantages over lettuce and other Western greens. Seaweeds are high in dietary iron, and they can help fight anemia, especially in women. It provides you with Magnesium, B vitamins, calcium, iodine and vitamin C. There many different types of seaweeds out there and if you are looking to break out from your boring vegetable routine, try some seaweed in your next salad. You may be pleasantly surprised.

Tofu

Tofu is actually an awesome food. It's like a blank canvas that inspired vegetarian chefs to create a multitude of dishes from. The best thing about tofu is its protein. Your steak and this sticky white stuff have the same amount of body building amino acids. The difference is that tofu has cholesterol lowering agents such as omega-3 fatty acids. It is also extremely high in calcium which can help older adults avoid the process of osteoporosis.

How does it taste? Well, for some it is an acquired taste. For some people, this stuff can taste like a juicy hamburger. For others, it can taste like that paste you ate in first grade. As with most vegetarian foods, it's all about how you prepare it. Fortunately, there are many products in the market that use tofu as a meat substitute. Try tofu burgers or tofu hot dogs. They are out there, they taste great, and they are healthier for you.

Vegetarian foods are among some of the healthiest foods out there. Exchange one vegetable dish for a seaweed concoction, eat tofu instead of steak at one meal per week, and work in some quinoa into your lifestyle. Your body will thank you and you may find that these "substitutes" are pretty appetizing in their own right.

EIGHT FOODS TO SLOW DOWN AGING

You think food can't help you live longer? Below is a list of eight foods that help you slow down aging:

Organic Eggs

Eggs contain all nine essential amino acids and include on average of about six grams of protein. Proteins are essential to the building, maintenance and repair of our skin, internal organs, muscles and are also an important component in keeping a healthy immune system and balanced hormones.

Make sure they are true organic free range and eat the whole egg to preserve all the nutrients.

Should You Eat Just the Egg White?

An egg's yolk contains roughly 150-180 milligrams of cholesterol. Many years ago cholesterol coming from foods was thought to be the major cause of unhealthy blood cholesterol, therefore egg yolks have been demonized and health nuts sticked to eating strictly egg whites.

Today we know that the real threat to high cholesterol is saturated and trans fats, not dietary cholesterol.

On the other hand, all the fat of the egg is stored in the yolk, the egg white contains no fat. This becomes only an issue though if you are eating a lot of eggs, for example when using eggs as a protein source for bodybuilding.

In summary: When you eat only the egg whites, you're missing out on half of the nutritional benefits and on half of the protein – but you are saving 100% of the fat.

Should You Eat Raw Eggs?

Some people choose to eat raw eggs because some nutrients can be diminished by heating. However, there is increased risk of salmonella infection in raw eggs. Cooking eggs until both the white and yolk are solid will kill any bacteria, such as salmonella.

The general consensus is that there is no significant advantage in eating eggs raw. Just because it's disgusting doesn't make it good for you.

2. Whey Protein

Whey protein has shown to increase your body's stores of glutathione — an antioxidant that increases the integrity of telomeres (bundles of DNA found in our cells).

Telomeres shorten as we age due to damages made by free radicals. The effects are aging and the start of age-related diseases such as Alzeimer's. Because of the effects of glutathione on the telomeres, glutathione has even been called "the master antioxidant."

The overall top food for maximizing your glutathione is high quality whey protein. By the way, exercise boosts your glutathione levels as well!

3. Broccoli

Broccoli is an antioxidant rich vegetable. It is high in isothiocyanates, a cancer fighting compound.Isothiocyanates have been shown to be especially effective in fighting lung and esophageal cancers. Other studies have shown that risks of other cancers of the gastrointestinal tract and the respiratory tract can be reduced by consuming isothiocyanate-rich vegetables.

Other foods that contain this compound are cauliflower, brussels sprouts, cabbage and horseradish. Try adding these types of vegetables to your weekly diet to lower the risk of lung, bladder and prostate cancer.

4. Leafy Greens

Kale, spinach, turnip greens, romaine lettuce and collard greens are rich in antioxidants that can reduce your risk of age related muscle degeneration, non-hodgkin's lymphoma and age-related short term memory loss. Try to eat naturally grown fresh vegetables.

Dark leafy greens are also high in vitamin K, which is linked to improved vascular health.

5. Chlorella

This is a single-celled fresh water algae plant. It contains vitamin C and carotenoids, both of which are antioxidants, as well as high concentrations of iron and B-complex vitamins. The health benefits are many, including:

- increases energy levels
- boosts immune system
- improves digestion
- improves concentration and ability to focus
- helps to balance PH levels
- may reduce risks of cancer because of the high vitamin density

The most important property of chlorella is its ability to help the body get rid of heavy metals toxins which can compromise your health. Look for a reputable brand of chlorella to get the best quality.

6. Blueberries

So yummy and so healthy, blueberries are full of antioxidants. The anthocyanins in blueberries help the brain to produce dopamine, which can improve your mood, co-ordination and memory. Eat a handful of blueberries a day and you reduce your risks of cancer, heart disease, short term memory loss, infections and many other ailments. Other berries that have these properties are cherries, blackberries, strawberries, cranberries and açaí berries.

7. Garlic

The component in garlic, which gives it that unique smell and taste, is allicin. When this is digested, it produces sulfenic acid, a compound that neutralizes free radicals faster than any other compound out there. Garlic has antibacterial, antifungal and antiviral properties too so it can helps fight infections, viruses and parasites. It can also enlarge blood vessels and improve blood flow especially to the heart which could prevent high blood pressure, heart attacks and strokes.

Garlic can also prevent cholesterol from becoming oxidized (which we don't want since the testes convert cholesterol into the prized hormone testosterone!) So eat fresh garlic because it can protect your body from prostate, colon and esophageal cancers and so many other ailments.

In order to get the full health benefits of garlic, use only fresh varieties and chop it or crush it. Wait a few minutes before eating it, but don't leave it for more than an hour.

8. Fish

The omega-3 in fish has anti-inflammatory properties which are vital in keeping brain tissues in good and healthy condition. Stick with relatively small fish like sardines, mackerel and wild salmon while limiting your consumption of tuna and swordfish as they have higher concentration of mercury. If fish is not your thing, try a good reputable brand of omega-3 supplement.

INTERMITTENT FASTING

Intermittent fasting (IF) is a pattern of eating that alternates between periods of fasting (usually meaning consumption of water and sometimes low-calorie drinks such as black coffee) and non-fasting.

So this means that Intermittent Fasting is not a diet per se, but an eating pattern, designed to improve health and longevity. Despite the marketing hype surrounding Intermittent Fasting, the research is still in its infancy – but it shows some promising benefits.

Intermittent Fasting Regimes

There are three popular fasting methods:

The 5:2 method. With this regime, you are not limited in your calorie intake for five days of the week but restrict your calorie intake to 400-600 calories per day for two days.

Alternate Day Fasting (ADF). ADF requires that you eat what you want on one day and keep your intake below 600 calories the following day.

The Lean Gains method. Basically, you skip breakfast. Men fast for 16 hours each day and women for 14 hours .For example, if your last meal is at 8pm tonight, you wouldn't eat again until 10am (women) or 12pm (men) tomorrow. During fasting you may only consume water or other non-caloric beverages.

How Does Intermittent Fasting Supposedly Work?

The main idea is that during fasting, the body is more likely to pull energy from stored fat, rather than the glucose in your blood stream or glycogen in your muscles/liver.

Fasting induces a cellular stress response (similar to that induced by exercise) in which cells up-regulate the expression of genes that increase the capacity to cope with stress and resist disease and aging.

Growth hormone production is increased during fasting, while insulin production is reduced. Increased insulin sensitivity retards aging and diseases that are associated with loss of insulin sensitivity, such as Type II Diabetes. This makes a workout supposedly more effective at both muscle building and fat loss after fasting.

What Does The Research Say?

Most of the Intermittent Fasting research has centered on IGF-1, a protein produced by the liver when it is stimulated by growth hormones circulating in the blood. High levels of IGF-1 are believed significantly to increase the risks of colorectal, breast and prostate cancer. Low levels of IGF-1 reduce those risks. It turns out that IGF-1 levels can be lowered by what you eat and this outcome has several benefits attached to it, especially for adults in their 40s.

Researchers from the University of Copenhagen, Denmark, suggest that fasting every other day provides the body with enough stress to activate the SIRT1 gene — which is linked to insulin sensitivity that leads to cellular release of fat into the bloodstream for use as energy by the muscles.

Research by Mark Hartman and colleagues indicates short-term fasting can trigger production of human growth hormone (HGH) in men, and reduce oxidative stress that contributes to disease and aging; benefits brain health, mental well-being, and clarity of thought.

Now, most of these effects have been demonstrated as well with other diets that reduce the calorie intake.

Potential Side Effects of Intermittent Fasting

At this time, little is known about possible side effects. Anecdotal reports of effects include:

- sleeping difficulties
- bad breath (a known problem with low carbohydrate diets)
- irritability
- anxiety
- daytime sleepiness

Intermittent Fasting is not advised for pregnant women and people with insulin-related health conditions, such as diabetes.

Remember to consult a registered dietician or physician before undertaking drastic changes in your diet.

So What's The Conclusion?

We think there are three points to keep in mind:

Intermittent Fasting is an eating pattern, not a diet. What you eat, the quantity and quality of foods, is still more important than when you eat it.

If you have issues with portion control or any other eating disorders, Intermittent Fasting is not for you.

If you are healthy, try it! What may work for one person may not work for another, because of differences in lifestyle, habits and genetics. Keep in mind that you don't have to follow any regimen strictly to the point. For example, to enhance your insulin sensitivity, try delaying or skipping breakfast.

If you're losing fat and not feeling hungry or lethargic, then continue with what you're doing!

THE DONT'S OF A HEALTHY LIFESTYLE

Who doesn't want to have a healthy lifestyle? Everybody does, so keep reading...

We are constantly bombarded with television commercials, print advertising, diet books, diet gurus and enough home fitness equipment to open up our very own gym. What is a would-be dieter really to do? What should you believe?

Well, this chapter is about the things you are not supposed to do if you want to live a healthy lifestyle.

Severe Caloric Restriction

You've got to eat. Far too many people make the mistake of restricting their calories too severely. Your body requires fuel to simply function and also to support your exercise program. If you deprive your body of adequate nutrition, your body will turn to other sources (like lean muscle tissue) for fuel. Failing to eat enough will probably cause you to lose weight, but you'll lose fingernails, hair and bone density as well.

Too Heavy Cardiovascular Exercise

You've seen the men and women at the gym who are draped over the Stairmaster. Hair matted down, shirt soaking wet and an unmistakable aura of desperation. If you cannot finish your cardio workout with proper form, you need to tone down the intensity or the length. Draping oneself over a cardio machine or clutching onto the guardrails for dear life is not recommended, nor is it a good workout.

Skipping Strength Training

Women are especially guilty of this one. Muscle tissue requires more calories to maintain itself than fatty tissue does. Strength training builds muscle. Therefore, if you increase the amount of lean muscle tissue, you will be able to eat more! Isn't that beautiful? Additionally, weight-bearing exercises are critical for bone health. If you aren't sure about form, hire a personal trainer for a session or two to get you started.

Skipping Meals

This one goes hand-in-hand with severe calorie restriction. Think about it... if you skip breakfast in an effort to lessen your calorie intake, you will be positively ravenous by lunchtime and much more likely to overeat. However, if you've had breakfast and a small snack, your hunger levels and blood sugar will be stable. This is why fitness professionals keep advocating smaller meals. Eating frequently throughout the day will keep both hunger and grouchiness at bay.

Taking Magic Fat Burning Pills

If you haven't actually purchased any, you may have at least picked them up in the grocery store. It is tempting and that little voice inside your head could be saying, "What if THIS ONE really works?" The most logical thing to do is step away from this magic fat burning pills. Take comfort in knowing that magic fat burning pills are nothing but a bunch of long marketing words strung together by a supplement company in the hope of making money. Rest assured that if there really WERE magic fat burning pills, we'd all look like supermodels.

Jumping on the Latest Diet Bandwagon

Anyone can drink shakes/abandon bread/eat cabbage soup/drink a shot of pineapple juice before and after each meal for at least a couple weeks. But come on, folks. This is about a lifestyle change. We all know that diet fads are fleeting and once we stop the trend, old habits re-emerge and we're back to square one.

Weight loss requires a lifestyle change and it's got to be doable. It's absolutely fine to follow guidelines, but look for plans that follow a reasonable and balanced approach. If you tilt your head and say "Really?" upon reading that banana is a fruit that cures all diseases, that ought to tell you something.

There is actually a silver bullet for weight loss – it's called common sense. Does it seem odd that diet gurus are telling you to never eat another piece of bread for as long as you live? Does it seem strange that a company would promise amazing results inside of a tiny white capsule? It should. If something makes you think twice, there's probably good reason for it.

Balance and moderation. It's boring. It's not sexy. But that's it right there. And you don't even need a book or a pill or a pantry stocked with low carb bread.

GOOD LUCK AND TO YOUR HEALTH

That is it from me! I hope you will enjoy your Green Juice Detox. It is a great starting point on your journey to be in shape, strong, and healthy.

From here on out, it is up to you to do the work to make the dream a reality (yes, you actually have to do some work).

Just remember to never let go of the dream and keep working every day towards your goal.

To your health!
Natalia Krasnyanskaya
www.top.me